THE
PAIN-FREE
KNEE
How to Have a Healthy, Happy Knee... Surgery-Free

DR. BRANT KOENIG, DC

ISBN Paperback: 978-0-578-52433-7

Acknowledgement

To quote Isaac Newton, "If I have seen further than others, it is by standing upon the shoulders of giants." Dr. Singer has been the giant upon whose shoulders I've stood throughout my career. Thank you for your guidance and teaching.

Chapter 1

Yes! You Can Have Pain-Free Knees without Surgery!

A patient of ours in his early sixties owned a small-town grocery store. It was a seven-day-a-week, labor-intensive business where he was constantly in motion—up and down, back and forth, in and out. He was unloading and stocking shipments, putting up and tearing down displays, building, repairing, cleaning, and certainly helping customers. He was the entire business.

But he had a problem: he suffered from chronic, debilitating knee pain—the kind of pain that curtailed his mobility and threatened his livelihood. He needed help fast.

He drove two hours to come to our clinic for stem cell injections and platelet-rich plasma, or PRP, injections. The result? He is now pain-free and fully functioning again. He's able to keep his business running optimally and participate in family, church, and community activities that he had missed out on because of his constant pain. He said his improvement made him "feel like a lizard that grew a new tail."

The myth about knee (and back) pain is that surgery is inevitable, the only choice. People may not know to explore other avenues for relief when their primary-care physician sends them to a surgeon who immediately advises them to undergo knee replacement—or they believe they should wait until they can't stand the pain anymore, and then have the surgery. What else can they think?

"Even if you don't do it now," they're told, "when you're older, you'll have the operation anyway because there are just no alternatives."

That can't be further from the truth.

There are alternatives that not only substitute for surgery, but also surpass it. In so many cases, these options provide complete pain relief and increased mobility with decreased recovery time.

Recovery time from knee or back surgery is up to three to six months and includes intensive, potentially painful rehabili-tation. There are also many instances when the surgery fails and the patients are left in as much pain as they were before the surgery—or they end up worse.

Cost savings is another positive component of surgery alternatives. The average knee replacement costs $49,500, and many of us have high insurance deductibles. Compound that by all the time spent away from work, and you have a formula for distress—not success. The options that you will read in this book can not only save you money, but also the pain and suffering of invasive surgery.

Let's look inside your knee and figure out why it seems to be subjected to all that pain and injury.

THE HUMAN KNEE

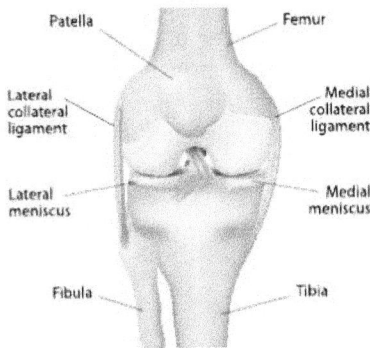

Patella — Femur

Lateral collateral ligament — Medial collateral ligament

Lateral meniscus — Medial meniscus

Fibula — Tibia

Bordered by the femur bone on top and the tibia on the bottom, the knee is the largest joint in the human body. It also is considered the most complicated one. The knee is comprised of the meniscus, the medial collateral ligament, lateral liga-ment, and patella (see diagram). The knee also contains the anterior cruciate ligament, or ACL, and posterior cruciate ligament. The knee joint is surrounded by a joint capsule, lined internally by a mucous membrane that produces *synovial fluid*, also known as *synovia*. Synovial fluid is like WD-40 for your joints. It must be present in sufficient quantity in the required consistency—just like a bike chain must always be well lubricated so that nothing squeaks.

Among the most common knee injuries is one that affects the ACL. Statistics show that one in every 3,500 people injures this ligament—a total of 100,000 to 200,000 incidents per year.[1] A lot of athletes suffer ACL injuries.

Because knees are extremities, on a daily basis they may be exposed to more trauma than other areas of the body. How many times have you bumped your knee while getting into or out of your car? As children, it's common to fall off a swing or bike and onto our knees. As we become elderly, falling becomes even more common (more on that later), and the knee is often the place where a falling person lands.

The fact that we always use our knees is no small matter. Every time we sit, stand, walk, squat, or run, we require our knees to perform. They absorb a lot of stress. In high school, college, and pro football, if an athlete is tackled from the side with the knee slightly bent—or if someone collides with the player on the basketball court, baseball diamond, or soccer field—any impact with the knee can cause injury, often to the ACL, mentioned previously. But not only athletes have knee problems. Each time you jump up and down or twist around—in a cardio class at the gym, for example—you risk injury. It's even possible to tear the meniscus—the fibrous cartilage that lines the knee joint.

Did you have surgery for an injury years ago? Chances are, there is arthritis developing around that joint now. In fact, some studies report that, even if you did what was considered the right thing by having surgery, you might develop arthritis faster than if you'd never had an injury. Many people manage their arthritic pain with medication and wait until it is unbearable, then opt for knee-replacement surgery. But surgery is not a guarantee of result and often has a high failure rate. Did you know that a frequent reason for surgery is prior surgery? Of course, with arthritis, age also has a lot to do with it. Many patients say, "Getting old is hell!" but I am here to present to you that getting old doesn't have to be hell.

With aging, our bodies slow down and change, resulting in weaker connections by way of muscles, joints, and bones. Cartilage—a smooth, resilient, elastic tissue—is a rubber-like padding that covers and protects the ends of long bones at the joints. Healthy cartilage is like a sponge: During compres-sion, metabolic products are squeezed outward, and during relaxation, nutrients can go inward. Cartilage is nourished in this way, since it is not supplied by blood vessels. But cartilage can be damaged and can wear away as we age.

You may accept the aging process, and you might even accept that surgery and medication are the only options to restore your function—but I am writing this book to tell you that they are *not* the only options. For example, stem cell therapy—a hallmark of our practice—can help regrow or repair the damaged joint space, ligaments, and meniscus.

Knee-Pain Perils

Knee surgery can have long-lasting side effects. Following surgery, in addition to a dearth of cartilage, knee space between the knee's components lessens, or degenerates. This may be become more apparent as people age. Diminished joint space can cause pain, immobility, and possibly falls due to instability.

Falling is an increasingly large problem in the elderly. According to the Centers for Disease Control and Prevention and National Council on Aging:
- One in four Americans aged sixty-five or older falls each year.
- Every eleven seconds, an older adult is treated in the emergency room for a fall. Every nineteen minutes, an older adult dies from a fall.
- Falls are the leading cause of fatal injury and the most common cause of nonfata,l trauma-related hospital admis-sions among older adults.

- Falls result in more than 2.8 million injuries treated in emergency departments annually, including more than 800,000 hospitalizations and 27,000 deaths.
- In 2013, the total cost of fall injuries was $34 billion.

- The financial toll for older-adult falls is expected to increase as the population ages, and may reach $67.7 billion by 2020.[2]

We all have heard of someone elderly who fell and died from complications of the fall. The way I see it, a fall in an older patient can be the beginning of the end. A close friend was in his seventies and lived a very active life, running his business full time until he hurt his knee, at which point his activity level went way down. In fact, he was rather immobile for three to four months. During this time, his immune system became depressed and he developed leukemia. There are many who believe in a mind-body connection, and this was clearly an example. This man underwent chemotherapy, which took its toll on his body. He died after a yearlong battle —and it all started with knee pain.

While not all knee injuries and pain will end this way, waiting until the pain is unbearable to tackle a knee issue with surgery is not the best course of action. The story of my friend may be an extreme case, but we see many patients who have accepted lives with pain as the "norm" because they have been in pain for so long. Many of them don't even remember life without knee pain. They're just sitting it out until their orthopedists tell them it's time for surgery.

I'm not saying surgery is unwarranted in all cases, but there are alternatives that many doctors are either unaware of or in which they are uninterested. Doctors may lack education in and experience with different modalities, and in some cases, it may be about economics. With the average knee-replacement surgery costing about $49,500, and a partial knee-replacement surgery costing just 10 to 20 percent less, the economics of practicing medicine is a consideration for the profession.

Skirting the Scalpel

In 2013, the *New England Journal of Medicine* reported on a Finnish study involving 146 patients, ages thirty-five to sixty-five, who needed arthroscopic partial meniscectomies— surgery to repair a degenerative meniscal tear, which is the most common orthopedic procedure performed in the United States. According to the *NEJM*, approximately 700,000 arthroscopic partial meniscectomies are performed annually in the United States, at a cost of an estimated $4 billion dollars.

After providing informed consent, about half of the group underwent the actual procedure, while the other half underwent placebo surgery—or as the report labeled it, "sham surgery."

The study's conclusion stated the following:

The results of this randomized, sham-controlled trial show that arthroscopic partial medial meniscectomy provides no significant benefit over sham surgery in patients with a degenerative meniscal tear and no knee osteoar-thritis. These results argue against the current practice of performing arthroscopic partial meniscectomy in patients with a degenerative meniscal tear.[3]

Think about that. Arthroscopic knee surgery had *no better results* than sham surgery!

One of the driving forces behind my writing this book is my sixty-six-year-old mother. As an active senior, she runs her business full time and exercises, including taking dance classes. One day, she heard a "pop" in her knee—and then suddenly, she couldn't walk. Without wanting to burden me, she went to her regular doctor, who prescribed pain medica-tion. A week or two went by, and her knee pain continued with little or no improvement. Her doctor referred her to an orthopedic specialist who told her she'd injured her meniscus. He told her it wasn't "that bad," but that because of her age, she already had some arthritis. He advised her he could clean it out arthroscopically, and when the time came, she could get knee-replacement surgery.

While her own daughter works at a clinic where knee pain is treated successfully without surgery, my mother suffered with debilitating knee pain for weeks—all because she did not want to bother me. I was shocked to discover she was considering surgery. I tell you, sometimes (or often!) your own family members make the most difficult patients.

I started my mother on a series of PRP (platelet-rich plasma) injections while supporting her knee with an appropriate knee brace. A number of athletes, including Tiger Woods, Kobe Bryant, and Alex Rodriguez, have reaped the benefits of PRP therapy (see Chapter 5). My mother also received knee-decompression therapy, which opened up the degenerative knee joint. In addition, stem cell injection regrew the knee space.

Within three weeks, she was walking, working, and dancing as if nothing had happened. She now tells me how her friends with knee injuries that happened years ago still can't walk right. They wonder how my mother is back to normal in such a short period of time.

Sometimes patients ask if genetics affect how strong and resilient our knees are. Genetics influences many things, disease among them. If arthritis runs in your family, you might develop arthritis. That doesn't mean you *will* get arthritis. It's not etched in stone that the gene will be expressed, but you may be predisposed to it in a way that someone who comes from a family where arthritis is not present won't. The science of epigenetics studies how environment affects genes. The studies of epigenetics tell us that your environment and your lifestyle can decide whether your gene will be pressed or not. So whether you will or won't experience disease and pain is not a hard-and-fast rule—even if many family members have that ailment.

Weighing In

One of the big factors in chronic knee pain is an individual's weight, which can be a result of genetics or environment—but it can also be caused by overeating, or just eating the wrong foods. When you're overweight—which statistics tell us 80 percent of Americans are—your body experiences inflamma-tion. I'm not talking about when a cut becomes infected and temporarily inflamed or when you sprain your ankle and it swells up immediately. The type of inflammation I'm referring to is a low-grade, chronic condition that results in pain and stiffness—which might make you more prone to injury because your joints don't move as well—and arthritic degeneration. Symptoms of low-grade inflammation may include difficulty losing weight, headaches, joint pain, and brain fog. You might develop a skin rash that won't go away. Low-grade inflammation also has been cited as a cause of heart disease.[4]

Many medical experts strongly believe the root of all disease is inflammation, so it is important to take steps to get inflam-mation under control. This can include an appropriate diet (avoiding certain foods that are known to cause or contribute to inflammation), exercise, and weight loss. While we want to treat everyone who comes to our clinic with highly effective alternatives to surgery, reducing overall inflammation of the body can make a big difference in improving the treatment's effectiveness and longevity.

Sources including WebMD report the benefits of weight loss may be multiplied fourfold for people who suffer from osteoarthritis, an inflammatory process which progressively destroys the cartilage. Again, cartilage acts as a shock absorber in the knee. One study showed that each pound of body weight lost resulted in a four-pound reduction in knee-joint stress.[5] Losing ten pounds means forty fewer pounds per step that your knees have to carry. It only makes sense that helping a patient lose excess weight when he or she comes in with knee pain will result in a better outcome.

Mastering Machines

If you are inclined to use a machine that exercises the knee without first addressing the cause of your knee pain, you may find yourself in trouble. The vast majority of knee-rehabilitation machines are designed to restore range of motion for people who've recently had arthroscopic or knee-replacement surgery. Others are just standard leg exercisers for thigh muscles like the quads and hamstrings, or for calf strengthening. These machines are not designed to work the knee, and certainly not to randomly exercise a painful, injured, degenerative knee.

That said, when knee spaces become jammed and arthritic, decompression therapy is a recommended course of action. Knee decompression is achieved with special motorized therapeutic equipment we have that gently—nonsurgically—opens up closed knee space to achieve optimal results. We mentioned earlier that the knee is filled with a lubricating, cushioning fluid: the synovial fluid. But this fluid cannot circulate if there is no space for it to do so. Knee decompression allows fluid to perform its function in the knee as it did presurgery, pre-injury, or prior to age-related issues.

Sometimes patients will come to me and say that one (if not both) of their knees is "bone on bone," meaning all protective cushioning has been lost. If they are really in that condition, it is generally impossible to walk or bend the knee without excruciating pain, or buckling, or falling, or all of the above—yet they walk into the office and sit in chair with their knees bent. The reason why I point this out is because even in the patients who were told they are bone on bone, we still find some joint space. For these patients, we employ a combination of knee decompressor, stem cell injections, natural supplements, and rehabilitation. The treatment works, with a consistently high success rate. In the face of impending surgery—which these "bone on bone" patients are told is their only option—it's certainly worth trying natural, less painful, and quicker-acting alternatives for healing. For the record, our oldest patient was ninety-two years old and had endured years of painful knee issues that we were able to resolve.

Another substance that has been quite successful in rejuve-nating knees is a specific hyaluronic acid injection. Hyaluronic acid is a substance made from collagen. Some patients call it a "rooster comb shot" because certain hyaluronic acid is derived from rooster comb. Collagen is the primary structural protein and the most abundant protein in our bodies. It is found in skin and other connective tissue, including muscles, bones, blood vessels, tendons, and the digestive system. You might see collagen advertised in commercial cosmetic products (in small amounts) and it is widely used in cosmetic procedures (in much larger amounts). Collagen, which is found naturally in the fluid that cushions and lubricates knee joints, helps with healing and repair. Injecting hyaluronic acid into an arthritic knee is like applying WD-40 to an old hinge. When used in conjunction with knee decompression, it can give the patient long-lasting relief.

Moving Images

It's hard to believe, but sometimes doctors who perform various forms of injections do not use any live imaging. They may refer to a previous x-ray or ultrasound. Many doctors do not use any imaging while they administer the injection. In our office, we use fluoroscopy.

Fluoroscopy is a study of moving body structures, similar to an x-ray "movie." A continuous beam is passed through the body part being examined or treated. The beam is transmitted to a monitor so that the body part and its motion can be seen in detail, like a video.

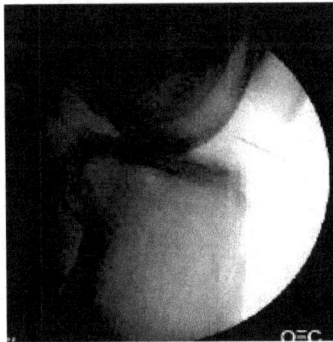

As an imaging tool, fluoroscopy enables physicians to look at many body systems, including the skeletal, digestive, urinary, respiratory, and reproductive systems.[6] In our practice, we use it to guide the needle with stem cells, PRP, or Hyalgan® (hyaluronic acid) to precisely where it needs to be in the knee without guesswork—and without having to rely on a still image that may be one-dimensional or months old.

Why Act Now?

Some patients will come in after having suffered with knee pain for weeks or months; others have been in pain for years. They might report that they've been unable to climb the stairs in their homes, or maybe they didn't go on that long-anticipated cruise with their spouse because they knew they just couldn't enjoy it. They can no longer walk the dog and are putting on weight, and perhaps they even sat out that special trip with their grandkids to Disney.

In the same vein, we also see a lot of patients with back pain, as well as neck and other joint pain. Sometimes issues can be interrelated. Repeatedly compensating for a bad knee can change one's posture, causing back pain—and conversely, a back that's out of whack can put undue pressure on the knees. Old injuries, such as a herniated disc, can still be painful because of degeneration and inflammation. Back pain can often be controlled by one or more of the same treatment modalities we practice. Although we do not give injections into the spine at our practice, we may refer patients to facilities that do so.

Optimally functioning knees are an essential component of good health. Pain and immobility affect our physical and emotional states, and, consequently, how we relate to our fami-lies, friends, and work. Healthy knees can mean the difference between a rich, fulfilling life and one that is lived incompletely. Ask someone who has spent months or years incapacitated by limited mobility and pain that does not subside. Pain might decrease for a few hours with the use of narcotics or other temporary pain relievers, which we will address in Chapter 2, but then the pain returns.

There is relief. There is a more permanent solution. We practice it every day!

[1] Friedberg, MD, Ryan P., "Anterior Cruciate Ligament Injury." UpToDate. March 20, 2017. http://www.uptodate.com/contents/anterior-cruciate-ligament-injury

[2] National Council on Aging. Undated. https://www.ncoa.org/news/resources-for-reporters/get-the-facts/falls-prevention-facts/

[3] Sihvonen, MD, Raine. "Arthroscopic Martial Meniscectomy versus Sham Surgery for a Degenerative Meniscal Tear." New England Journal of Medicine. December 26, 2013. http://www.nejm.org/doi/full/10.1056/ NEJMoa1305189#t=article

[4] Inflammation and Heart Disease. American Heart Association. October 12, 2016. http://www.heart.org/HEARTORG/Conditions/Inflammation-and-Heart-Disease_UCM_432150_Article.jsp#.WPUQVojyvIU

[5] Jennifer Warner. Small Weight Loss Takes Big Pressure off Knee. WebMD. June 29, 2015. http://www.webmd.com/osteoarthritis/news/20050629/ small-weight-loss-takes-pressure-off-knee

[6] Fluoroscopy Procedure. Johns Hopkins Medicine Health Library. Undated. http://www.hopkinsmedicine.org/healthlibrary/test_procedures/orthopaedic/ fluoroscopy_procedure_92,P07662/

Chapter 2

There's No Magic Pill for Knee Pain—But You Already Knew That

It's true. There is no magic pill for knee pain, and to try and alleviate pain and fix the problem with a single drug—or multiple drugs, as some people do —may be not only futile, but also dangerous. And I'm not only talking about the kind of drugs that cause dependence, which we'll explore later in this chapter.

In his book *Mind Over Meds*, integrative medicine physician Dr. Andrew Weil writes that overmedicating is a serious issue in this country. Based on the number of drugs Americans are taking, there is increased risk of adverse drug reactions—some-thing Dr. Weil claims is among the leading causes of death.[7]

Dr. Pieter Cohen, Harvard Medical School Assistant Professor of Medicine and General Internist at Cambridge Health Alliance in Somerville, Massachusetts, has admitted, "We under-perceive the risks of those medications we prescribe."[8]

Polypharmacy—defined as the simultaneous use of multiple drugs by an individual for one or more conditions—is a signifi-cant problem in the United States. Statistics tell us substance abuse and addiction cost taxpayers hundreds of billions of dollars a year, not to mention the personal, family, workplace, community, and societal toll these issues take.

But let's start with nonsteroidal anti-inflammatory drugs (NSAIDs). Many pain medicines fall into the NSAIDs family. While NSAIDS are often not seen in the realm of abuse and addiction, we can come to rely heavily on them. Their purpose is to stop pain and reduce inflammation, which I've mentioned can be rampant in the body. Inflammation is a component of any knee-pain issue. But repeated use of NSAIDs can create a ticking time bomb.

Long-term use of NSAIDs, known by generic names that include aspirin, ibuprofen, acetaminophen, and naproxen—and commercially known as Motrin, Advil, and Aleve, to name a few—can cause harsh side effects, including irreparable kidney and liver damage.

Because knee pain is usually chronic, by the time they eventually seek us out—something I am trying to change by writing this book—many patients have been using NSAIDs for months or years. One of the deadly side effects of NSAIDs is the damage it does to kidneys. Some patients come in with stage 3 or 4 kidney failure from long-term use of NSAIDs medication. I remember one patient who cried through the whole consultation because he was just diagnosed with stage 4 kidney failure as a result of long-term NSAIDs use. No doctor had warned him about the danger of long-term pain medications and he felt failed by doctors.

NSAIDs can be effective in treatment of pain for short-term relief. They work to reduce the amount of *prostaglandin* your body makes. Prostaglandin, a natural substance produced by most cells and released when you sustain an injury, contributes to inflammation and causes a variety of effects including swelling, fever, and increased sensitivity to pain. By blocking your body's production of prostaglandins, NSAIDs can help reduce and relieve these symptoms of injury.[9] But their use is controversial because they also are known to cause nausea, vomiting, stomach bleeding, ulcers, diarrhea, constipation, loss of appetite, rash, headache, and drowsiness. As mentioned earlier, over time, they can also cause organ failure, especially failure of the kidney.

This category of drugs can also cause fluid retention (edema), manifested in the swelling of the ankles and legs.
NSAIDs can also cause prolonged bleeding after injury or surgery.[10] In 2015, a Harvard Medical School publication said experts have known for fifteen years that NSAIDs increase the risk of heart attack and stroke. They may also elevate blood pressure and cause heart failure. Some of the detailed warnings include:

- Heart attack and stroke risk increase even with short-term use, and the risk may begin within a few weeks of starting to take an NSAID.

· The risk increases with higher doses of NSAIDs taken for longer periods of time.

· The risk is greatest for people who already have heart disease, though even people without heart disease may be at risk.[11]

Here's another interesting fact: Though acetaminophen (brand name Tylenol) is not an NSAID—and therefore does not address inflammation—some people reach for it in their search for a painkiller. But in recent years, some studies have linked acetaminophen use to not just to a dulling of physical pain, but to a dulling of emotions as well! The explanation is, when the drug is ingested, the brain may not distinguish between your aching knee (or shoulder or a headache) and the emotional pain you are experiencing—even empathy for a friend. Studies have shown acetaminophen may compromise both bad and *good* emotions, causing us not to feel the levels of joy or excitement we might feel when not under the influ-ence of the drug, so to speak.[12] Of course, we want to get rid of physical pain—but do we really want to go through life masking or muting *all* emotions? There has to be a better, safer way to handle pain—and it's surely *not* steroids.

Another treatment doctors often recommend is steroids or cortisone to decrease inflammation and chronic pain. These may include oral steroids—prednisone/prednisolone, hydrocortisone, methylprednisolone, and others—or steroid injections. While steroids can be helpful in a short course to address a specific pain, continued use of oral steroids for chronic pain can carry daunting side effects.

Steroids (also known as cortisone or corticosteroids) are actually hormones that occur naturally in the body. These chemical messengers decrease inflammation but also suppress the body's immune system and block DNA from being made. They also block chemical called *histamine,* which is released during an allergic reaction. Steroid medicines are man-made, but they are chemically similar to these natural hormones.[13]

Unfortunately, prescription steroids, even when used for a short period of time, can cause symptoms of sleeplessness, anxiety, and increased hunger and thirst. Used for longer periods, steroids can lead to an increased risk of infection, because steroids work by suppressing the immune system. Steroid use can lead to high blood pressure, thinning and easily bruised skin, mood and behavioral changes, joint destruction (from injections), escalated risk of developing cataracts, and stomach or duodenal ulcers.

Weight gain is another common byproduct of oral steroid medication or injections. It's not unusual for me to see new patients who say they have gained forty or fifty pounds after being prescribed steroids. Often, their efforts to take off the excess weight are thwarted because the body's hormonal system is affected by having taken steroids—and as we've mentioned, if you have chronic knee (or back) pain, gaining weight puts added pressure on the joint, which will only compound the problem. What's more, the weight people tend to gain from steroids is around the middle—so-called "belly fat"—which is a known precursor to diabetes.

Along with weight gain, steroid injections also increase bone loss of up to 8 percent per injection. When a bone is viewed under a microscope after a steroid injection, it looks like acid has been poured on it. This is one of the reasons why many insurance companies allow only three steroid injections in a year—because repeated steroid injections will shorten the time needed before joint replacement, and joint replacement surgery is expensive for insurance companies. Continued steroid use can lead to osteoporosis, or thinning and weakening of the skeletal system.

At this point, I want to note the parameters within which many doctors must practice. Many are stuck recommending strictly what a managed health-care provider allows. It's not always what's best for the patient, but their hands are tied—for now, anyway—because treatments are dictated by our managed health-care system. Driven by profits, insurance policies are written to benefit the insurance company—not the patients or the physicians.

Unfortunately, patient care often comes down to the contract that the physician signed with the managed-care company for which he or she works

—or what the patient's insurance company will allow—and not what the doctor thinks will be best for the patient. I firmly believe doctors should be free to recommend what they believe is best for their patients, and patients should be free to choose what they know is best for them. Treatment options should be based on what doctors and patients know—not what the insurance company says is needed.

Abuse, Addiction, and America

It's not exactly breaking news that opioid abuse has reached epidemic proportions in this country. Drugs like OxyContin, hydrocodone, Valium, Vicodin, and others reportedly kill more people each year than illegal drugs.

Opioids are widely prescribed by doctors for chronic pain. In 2015, *Forbes* put the fortune of the Sackler family—whose company, Purdue Pharma, manufactures OxyContin, made from oxycodone—at $14 billion dollars. (In 2016, *Forbes* reported that number had dropped to $13 billion.)

Since OxyContin's launch in 1995, Purdue Pharma's overall sales have exceeded $35 billion dollars—mostly profits from prescriptions for OxyContin, which was developed that same year as an "addiction-proof" version of oxycodone. The Sack-lers, by way of information, also own separate drug companies that sell OxyContin and other drugs to Asia, Latin America, Canada, and Europe, together generating similar total sales as Purdue's operation in the United States.[14]

Though OxyContin is not the only culprit in skyrocketing levels of addiction, the history of this drug is an example of the wheels of economics that drive decision-making—in medicine as in other arenas. Patients sometimes pay a woeful price.

If a patient who has been chronically and habitually using prescription narcotics comes to us, we don't consider him or her a viable knee or back-pain therapy candidate. Under those circumstances, our treatments are likely to have a very high failure rate. These individuals typically need drug rehabilitation first, and we try and help them with referrals in that regard. Once they are free from drug dependence, we can reevaluate their condition and see if stem cell, PRP, decompression, and/ or other therapies, including Class 4 lasers (Chapter 7), our clinic provides can be helpful.

The Health Habit

Getting and staying healthy is our goal for patients. If patients are overweight—meaning there is certainly inflamma-tion—we put them on a thirty-day meal plan. The diet helps to detox their bodies. We also like to recommend supplements such as methylsulfonylmethane (MSM), a product found in glucos-amine that has virtually no side effects. MSM helps detoxify the body to some degree. Herbs including turmeric—used in mustard and available in supplement form, and curcumin—a chemical derived from plants —are also good for inflamma-tion. One of our patients, "Ray," came to us overweight and on six prescriptions, including Lyrica and others for pain. At the end of the thirty-day diet, he was off all of his meds and is completely pain-free. Exercise and nutrition are medicine and there can be no healing without them.

Many of our patients are also vitamin D deficient. This particular vitamin has an influence on every aspect of our health, including helping to control inflammation. Vitamin D is associated with bone density, helping to facilitate optimal calcium absorption. Prolonged deficiency of vitamin D can lead to rickets, a softening and weakening of the bones that was common in the old days, but unfortunately still affects people in some pockets of the country where extreme poverty exists. Inadequate vitamin D levels also impact immune system function and hormone production.

Although sun exposure can lead to skin cancer, the kind of vitamin D we acquire from the sun far exceeds what we can get from a bottle. Our bodies are designed to get the vitamin D they need from skin exposed to the sun. In fact, sunbathing used to be recommended as a legitimate form of treatment for achy joints and rheumatoid arthritis, before the advent of all kinds of pain medications.

I have firsthand experience with vitamin D deficiency. When I first started my clinic, I was working twelve-hour to thirteen-hour days. I'd arrive around dawn and often not leave until it was dark. By profession, I am a chiropractor, so I was adjusting lots of spines. I developed wrist pain I could not get rid of and knew there had to be inflammation associated with it.

At the time, I was also member of a coed soccer team. One day, we had a half-day practice right under the strong Houston sun. I played a few hours of soccer, went home, and the next morning my wrist pain was gone.

A simple blood test can tell whether a patient is getting enough vitamin D, and the solution might be a supplement or more sun exposure. While I don't endorse lying out and baking for hours on end, there is a lot to be said about what nature—and our own bodies—have to offer us in terms of healing. We just have to pay attention.

[7] Weil, Andrew. *Mind Over Meds: Know When Drugs Are Necessary, When Alternatives Are Better — and When to Let Your Body Heal on Its Own.* Little, Brown and Company. April 2017.

[8] Cohen, Pieter. "On Point." National Public Radio broadcast. May 3, 2017.

[9] "Is Aspirin an NSAID?" Healthline. Undated. http://www.healthline.com/ health/pain-relief/is-aspirin-nsaid#overview1

[10] Marks, MD, Jay W. and Ogbru, PharmD, Omudhome. "Nonsteroidal Inflammatory Drugs (NSAIDS)." MedicineNet. Undated. http://www.medicinenet.com/nonsteroidal_antiinflammatory_drugs/page2.htm
[11] Curfman, MD, Gregory. "FDA Strengthens Warnings That NSAIDs Increase Heart Attack and Stroke Risk." Harvard Health Publications. Harvard Medical

[12] "Tylenol: More Than Just a Pain Killer." Social Psychology Online. May 24, 2016. http://socialpsychonline.com/2016/05/tylenol-pain-psychology-acetaminophen/
School. http://www.health.harvard.edu/blog/fda-strengthens-warning-that-nsaids-increase-heart-attack-and-stroke-risk-201507138138
[13] "Oral Steroids." Patient. Undated. https://patient.info/health/oral-steroids
8.   [14] Morrell, Alex. "The OxyContin Clan: The $14 Billion Newcomer to Forbes 2015 List of Richest   U.S.   Families."   Forbes.   July   1,   2015.   https://www.forbes.com/sites/alexmorrell/2015/07/01/the-oxycontin-clan-the-14-billion-newcomer-to-forbes-2015-list-of-richest-u-s-families/#135b78c575e0

Chapter 3

Knee Pain and the Old West

Reward! Wanted Dead or Alive

The story goes that a wanted poster for a stagecoach robber got into the hands of a local sheriff. It also made its way around to the townsfolk, including a noted gunslinger.

Now, while some of us may think of a gunslinger as a man on the wrong side of the law, the dictionary tells us it's actually someone who carries a gun and shoots well. In a broader sense, a gunslinger is someone bold, assertive, and determined. There is surely something to be said for being quick on the draw—having the courage to pull the trigger while others are still in the gun store. And if you don't like gun analogies, let's just say there's something wise in making a quick, prudent decision—because over-deliberation can end up costing you a lot.

When word got out that the stagecoach robber might be on the outskirts of town, on the way to his next robbery, the gunslinger wasted no time; he looked over a map to decide upon his route, saddled up, and went after him. The sheriff, on the other hand, took a lot of time further analyzing the situation. He wired for more particulars, assembling just the right kind of posse and packing supplies, and choosing just the right horses.

The sheriff's group was just riding out as the gunslinger was returning—with the outlaw in hand (or actually in handcuffs).

No one is saying we shouldn't take some time to thoroughly investigate a situation. Jumping in blindly is seldom a good idea. We understand that sometimes people are nervous and apprehensive when they first come to see us. But there are instances when prospective patients tend to overdo it—even armed with a lot of material from our website, brochures, a consultation where one of our doctors spends an hour or more with them, and answers garnered from a first visit. They might put off the decision-making, prolonging their own pain and inconvenience and unnecessarily delaying important treatment.

"I just need more information," is a typical declaration, even after the individual has been provided with extensive research about different treatment options and our doctors have thor-oughly answered all of their questions. At that point, I generally ask what more they need—and how we can satisfy that.

"I just have to think about it," they say, over and over.

Suzanne (not her real name) came to our clinic just prior to her sixtieth birthday. Five years into the kind of pain from a knee injury that had curtailed both her work life and personal life. She had tried various medications prescribed by her doctor, plus remedies like heat and cold she randomly applied, and just about everything else she could think of—and none of it had helped. When she had to sit out a long-planned trip to Disney with her grandchildren, Suzanne decided it was the last straw. An acquaintance recommended our clinic. Still, she was wary at our first meeting.

"I've been having knee problems for years," she admitted. "I have to sit too much at work [she works in a department store] and have gone down to part time as a result. I need help around the house. I can't go for long bike rides or walks with my husband like we used to, and my stomach is constantly upset from the meds I take. Now my time with the grandkids is affected. But I'm still not sure about this."

Then she, as the saying goes, added insult to injury.

"You know, it's true I've had this condition for so long; it really would be great to get some relief," she said. "But then again, it doesn't bother me all *that* much. I'm almost used to it." She was talking herself into and out of, and again into and out of, treatment.

We understand it is human nature to be wary of the unknown, but minimizing what's really going on isn't in your best interest. At the same time, human beings have an innate ability to become so habituated to something that what's absolutely *not* normal (like pain and inconvenience) becomes the norm. This is part of a coping mechanism, and it can lead us to settle for far less than we should have to.

Just because you've had something for a long time doesn't make it normal or acceptable. Knee pain—or any kind of pain—simply isn't normal. Even though you may have endured and worked around it for years, you don't have to stay in pain—especially when there's a possible solution available. We use the example of a child complaining about an injury that has persisted. Would you tell that child that, because he or she has had this condition for the last few weeks, months, or years, he or she should "just learn to live with it?" Of course not! The same goes for you. Why would you consider your condition any different? Why would you not take care of yourself the way you would a child?

To take it one step further, if you don't take care of yourself, how will you be able to take care of anyone else? Some people (we find this a lot with female patients) are so busy doing things for others, they put their needs last. And though it may be a cliché to some extent, men are typically doctor-averse, making them accomplished at categorizing the pain they've had for years as "normal." We often hear about doctor-averse patients saying they're simply going to wait until the pain is so paralyzing, the dozens of medications they've tried have failed, and they cannot function at all—and then have surgery. What's five or ten more years, when you have already been suffering for that many?

If you are a "fact finder" patient, I hope this book serves as an excellent information source. I strive to thoroughly explain what we do to everyone, taking extra time to reassure prospec-tive patients who are entirely unfamiliar with our therapies of their merits.

That being said, not everyone is the right candidate for our clinic. While there are exceptions, over time, we've learned that the best patient for us is one who is either actively seeking different treatments or has truly reached the end of their rope with the pain and inconvenience their condition has caused. They may have exhausted any and all medications prescribed to resolve or lessen their pain, and/or the side effects have become unmanageable. Steroid injections no longer work. They come to the first appointment at least relatively informed about the kinds of therapies we provide, and we are pleased to go into greater detail and tailor a treatment plan to them. These patients are just plain sick and tired of living their lives short of their potential, and are ready to take the next step.

Sandra (also not her real name—all patient names have been changed) is a middle-aged patient of ours, a nurse who worked twelve-hour shifts with bilateral knee pain. By the second or third hour of each workday, she was already in pain, and by the fifth or sixth hour, it was often unbearable. She was afraid of losing her job or getting to the point where she simply could not walk because of the pain. After hearing about the platelet-rich plasma, or PRP, therapy our office offers (see Chapter 5), she came to us. She said she was sick and tired of dealing with her condition and was ready to do something about it. You might say Sandra was a gunslinger! We immediately started PRP therapy, along with knee decompression. Within about two weeks, her pain was completely gone. It was as though she'd never had it.

Everyone is different in terms of how they approach a situation, and we are not encouraging anyone to do some-thing that sends up a red flag for them. So much of healing is about attitude, and going into a procedure with faith and confidence in a positive outcome is half the battle. Just like most everything in life, being pain-free or getting healthy can start with one decision. You can continue to gather more and more information, and know everything else there is to know about it—but all that information and knowledge will mean nothing if you don't act on it. I encourage you to act on the information this book provides and try something different to treat your knee pain.

Chapter 4

Stem Cell Therapy: How to Turn Back the Clock for Your Knee

Stem cells have been called the "cellular putty" from which all tissues of the body are made. They are immature cells that have the ability to develop into many types of cells in your body. When applied to a degenerative, injured site, they rapidly work to support soft-tissue repair, reduce inflamma-tion, eliminate pain, minimize scar formation, and return lost function. Stem cells are the cornerstone of regenerative medicine.

Since 1981, when embryonic stem cells were first identified in mice, and especially since 1998 when they were first grown in a lab, researchers have dreamed of using these cells to repair damaged tissue or create new organs. [15] In fact, brushes with stem cells go all the way back to the 1960s when University of Toronto researchers, Dr. Earnest McCulloch and Dr. James E. Till, injected bone marrow into irradiated mice and observed the appearance of nodules, later determined to be stem cells capable of self-renewal, on their spleens.

Though the procedure is not without controversy, umbilical cord tissue stem cells have been used for years to successfully regenerate injured and compromised tissue. Umbilical cord stem cell tissues are different than embryonic stem cells and do not contain any fetal tissues. Using umbilical cord stem cells as a treatment protocol at Oklahoma Physical Medicine, sometimes in tandem with other treatments like platelet-rich plasma (PRP) therapy, which we'll discuss in the next chapter—or Class 4 lasers, which we'll describe in Chapter 6—we've seen tremendous results in regenerating degenerative joints.

When discussing stem cell therapy as a possible treatment option, one of the most frequently asked questions is, "Where do stem cells come from?"

There are three widely-used sources for stem cells:

- Bone marrow, which requires extraction by drilling into the bone
- Adipose tissue, which is lipid (or fat) cells, harvested by liposuction
- Umbilical cord tissue, or "waste products" of the birthing process," such as amniotic-tissue placenta—with stem cells taken just after birth—which we consider the apex of stem cell treatments

We will not consider other sources, such as embryonic stem cells, which are the subject of ongoing controversy. Embryonic stem cells are "totipotent," which means they have the ability to form into a whole new human being. The intention of this book is to facilitate *healing*, not to discuss *cloning*.

Should you decide to use stem cells from your own bone marrow, or from your adipose (fat) tissue, your stem cell quality declines the more you age. This is because the cells are affected by exposure over the years to pollution, pesticides, and other chemicals. Stem cells from adult bone marrow or adipose tissue will not be as helpful as those from umbilical cord tissue that is part of the birthing process.

The older you get, the worse the quality of your adult stem cells from bone marrow become. Stem cells from adults do not divide as fast as stem cells from umbilical cord tissue, and because of that, improvement is often not long lasting.

Additionally, in the process of harvesting stem cells from adipose tissue, cells must be treated with chemicals and enzymes—a process that can kill a lot of the precious stem cells. The number of active stem cells that can be harvested from a patient's own bone marrow or adipose tissue is about 1,600 —compared to umbilical cord tissue stem cells, which number one to three million.

What's more, stem cells from your bone marrow or adipose tissue will *differentiate*—a natural process in which one cell becomes two, two become four, four become eight and so on, resulting in regeneration and healing—for only about thirty days. Umbilical cord stem cells differentiate for more than 270 days. Which stem cells would you rather have working for you: those from your aging body or those from a new birthing process?

The umbilical cord tissue stem cells we inject into your knee can be on the job, repairing and regenerating tissue nine times longer than stem cells harvested from other sources. These *multipotent* stem cells can differentiate into many different tissues in the body. They can become hair cells, bone cells, or nerve cells. They can develop into most tissues or body parts.

In the (maybe not too distant) future, stem cells will essentially be medical miracles, used to eradicate diseases, including cancer, and to rejuvenate organs. If you have a heart defect, kidney failure, macular degeneration, a spinal-cord injury including paralysis, diabetes, Parkinson's disease, ALS, multiple sclerosis, muscular dystrophy, Alzheimer's disease, schizophrenia, autoimmune diseases (including lupus and rheumatoid arthritis), or lung or liver disease—or even if you need to regrow a tooth—the day is coming when you may be able to change or save your life with stem cells.

The unfortunate thing right now is that stem cells are in limited supply. These so-called "waste products" of the birthing process—such as umbilical cords, placenta, cord blood, and amniotic tissue—are usually discarded in hospital settings, when instead they could be used to help so many patients.

The umbilical cord tissue stem cells we use do their part to alleviate, if not completely eliminate, debilitating knee pain. Patients who have lived in chronic pain agree that living pain-free with improved function is already a medical miracle of sorts. What's more, the umbilical cord tissue stem cells we use come from an FDA-certified lab that must follow the rigorous standards and practices of the American Association of Tissue Banks (AATB). The donated tissues are screened, tested, and studied thoroughly following AATB's guidelines to make sure they are not contaminated with any pathogens that could potentially make you sick.

Administering the Healing

My mother, first mentioned in Chapter 1, experienced severe arthritis in her right hand because she did a lot of manual work. She could not fully close her hand, so we gave her two units of intravenous stem cells. While most of our stem cell therapy is directed to the source of the injury or pain by injection, in this case—because my mother has other issues, including diabetes, which has broken down her body quite a bit—we chose to administer the cells intravenously, trusting that stem cells and cytokines have the ability to find injured areas of the body and start the repair process.

As mentioned earlier in the chapter, when the body is injured and tissues need to regenerate, stem cells seem to *know* exactly where to go. This is achieved through a signal link system called the *cytokine network*. Within fifteen minutes, because my mother's hand was the part of her body giving her the most trouble, the stem cells had traveled there and she was able to close her hand much more than she had previ-ously been able to do. Over time, as the stem cells continued to differentiate, her hand improved even more. In imaging studies using radioactive dye, you can see that there are far more stem cells attracted to a patient's injured hand than to the unaffected hand.

If stem cells are injected into the knee with a compromised meniscus, for example, the cells will differentiate the meniscus from other parts. They will differentiate the synovial fluid, working to replenish and regrow tissue in the problematic knee space. What's also user-friendly about this type of stem cell therapy is that there's no downtime during which the body has to adjust to the treatment. Patients can get the injection and drive right home or back to work.

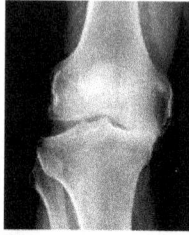

Knee before stem cell therapy

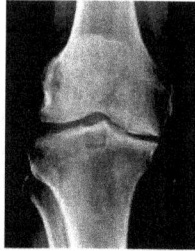

Knee after stem cell therapy

We do stress that, for optimal effect, it's important to stay away from sugar, gluten, and dairy for the first thirty days after a stem cell injection. These foods cause inflammation, and we don't want to impede the work that the stem cells are introduced to do. Some diabetic patients do not respond well to stem cell therapy because of their overall inflammation problems and poor circulation. For this reason, we put them on our preferred thirty-day meal plan, including the supplements referenced in Chapter 2, a month ahead of the procedure, and we ask them to stay away from sugar, gluten, and dairy afterward to encourage the best possible results.

As I write this book, I am excited about the future of medicine, especially where regenerative medicine is headed. The possibilities are limitless, and in addition to the kind of healing that is possible now, we'll soon be able to conquer many diseases that we previously couldn't cure.

---

[15] Coghlan, Andy. "Stem Cell Timeline: The History of a Medical Sensation." New Scientist. January 30, 2014. https://www.newscientist.com/article/ dn24970-stem-cell-timeline-the-history-of-a-medical-sensation/

Chapter 5

PRP: Heal Like the Pros!

Even if we can't quote chapter and verse about their latest birdie—or backhand smash, home run, or alley-oop—most of us know about great athletes like Tiger Woods, Maria Sharapova, Alex Rodriguez, and Kobe Bryant. But you may not know these elite athletes and many others of their ilks have one thing in common they have sought help for their pain and injuries with PRP injections as an alternative to surgery.

Surgery can sideline an athlete for weeks, months, or longer—and often, when a stellar RBI record succumbs to a nagging shoulder or knee injury, surgery just doesn't produce its intended results. Surgery can sideline us too, especially when weeks and months of recovery time (and pain) continue to interrupt our daily lives.

So what exactly is PRP, and why do we recommend it over surgery at our clinic?

PRP stands for platelet-rich plasma. Utilized since 1987, PRP is obtained by drawing a small amount of blood from the patient and spinning it in a centrifuge. This process separates infection-fighting white blood cells and the red blood cells that carry oxygen from the platelets and plasma. The platelets with the plasma have all of the body's healing agents. In fact, when you get a cut, it's the platelets that rush to the site and start the healing process.

Once the separation is completed, the platelet-rich plasma is concentrated. Activating materials are then added and the plasma is injected back into the patient—all within twenty to thirty minutes from the time blood was drawn. Because it is the patient's own platelet-rich plasma—not taken from a donor or synthesized in a laboratory[16]—there is no chance for rejection or risk of transmissible infection. Overall, PRP injec-tions are a considered a low-pain, low-risk procedure. There is no downtime. Most patients leave immediately afterward to resume their normal daily activities. The entire appointment at our clinic takes about an hour.

Platelets, which are blood's clotting cells, have the ability to induce healing in muscles, tendons, and ligaments. Growth factors released by platelets are said to recruit reparative cells, including the stem cells mentioned in Chapter 4, which augment tissue repair and accelerate soft-tissue healing. While we use this procedure to help repair knees and alleviate chronic pain, PRP has also been injected into spinal ligaments, facet joints, and/or intervertebral discs when traditional treatments have failed.[17] I recently read that some Major League Baseball players are using PRP injections as a preventative measure for shoulder, elbow, and wrist joints.

In my own office, I may use a combination of PRP and stem cell injections (which provide more than the PRP "recruited" stem cells mentioned above) to stimulate healing. The deci-sion to combine these protocols really depends on the level of degeneration, length of time the pain has persisted, and age of the patient.

For example, a younger person with a knee injury that's been plaguing him or her for a few weeks, or even a few months, will not have a great deal of degenerative, arthritic changes to the knee. Chances are we will successfully treat this individual strictly with PRP injections. If the patient is older, having suffered with chronic pain over a longer period of time—and if imaging shows us a great deal of degenerative change—he or she is often better off with stem cell injections. In many cases, a combination of PRP injections and stem cell injections can eliminate the pain by accelerating healing. The stem cells continue to differentiate over approximately 270 days (as mentioned in Chapter 4) to produce the best results.

At my clinic, based on the approximately five hundred patients who've received PRP injections to date, we've seen instant results and we've also seen it take two to four weeks to begin to work. Because we are helping the area to regen-erate, it's not a temporary fix. Most patients require a series of three to five PRP injections, but the result can be long lasting. Giving a PRP injection is equivalent to causing a rush of blood to promote healing, but without all the pain, swelling, and redness that occur when inflammation causes this rush of blood.

The only time PRP may not work is when a candidate has a platelet dysfunction, such as thrombocytopenia, hemo-dynamic instability, or other blood pressure issues (especially hypotension, i.e., low blood pressure). The procedure may be contraindicated if the candidate has active cancer or is currently undergoing cancer treatment, is taking a high dose of blood-thinning medication, or has metabolic disease. At our clinic, we evaluate patients and their conditions in terms of PRP-therapy eligibility in case-by-case reviews.

All About Bob

Bob was a patient in his mid-fifties who came to us after receiving steroid injections in his shoulder up to three times a year for several years. In the beginning, each injection would last months, and he was delighted; he was pain-free. But over time, he realized these injections were becoming less effective because steroid injection does not stop a degenerative joint condition. Eventually, he reached a point at which an injection would bring relief that lasted only a few days. What's more, he was concerned about the risks of repeated steroid use (which we discussed in Chapter 2).

Bob received a series of five PRP injections, along with Class 4 laser treatments (see Chapter 7). I ran into him in a grocery store a few years later. He gave me a big hug and reported that he was still pain free.

To reiterate, the therapies we recommend are contingent on the length of time someone has been experiencing pain, how much degeneration we see on imaging, an individual's age, and his or her state of health.

No Limits in Sight!

Doctors have been exploring the possibilities of PRP therapy for about twenty years, using it to repair injured heart muscles following heart failure or a heart attack, and to aid in the healing of sternal wounds when the sternum is opened for surgery. Studies have shown that patients heal better with the inclusion of PRP.[18][19]

Kim Kardashian has sung the praises of platelet-rich plasma facial rejuvenation, which works because PRP stimulates the production of collagen and elastin. She calls the procedure a "vampire facial" due to its blood component! The inventor of this procedure, Dr. Charles Runels, also invented O-Shot and P-Shot to help women and men achieve a more satisfying sex life. In addition, he invented other applications of PRP therapy, such as the PRP breast lift and PRP hair restoration. PRP seems like a fountain of youth for many parts of the body!

PRP might not be "magical," but it is a serious, highly effective therapy. The uses for PRP continue to expand along with medical science. While it's not a panacea for chronic pain, some patients tell us it comes pretty close.

If you've been living with pain for weeks, months, or years, and if your quality of life has been compromised due to diminishing joint function, PRP therapy might help return you to a pre-injury lifestyle and keep you there—if not forever, then for a very long time.

[16] "Patient Care. PRP Treatment Therapy. Platelet-Rich Plasma Therapy Speeds Healing of Musculoskeletal Injuries." Columbia University Medical Center. http://cses.cumc.columbia.edu/care-newtreatment.html

2. [17] "Platelet Rich Plasma (PRP)." Virginia Spine Institute. https://www.spinemd.com/treatments/platelet-rich-plasma

[18] "Evaluation of Autologous Platelet Rich Plasma for Cardiac Surgery: Outcome Analysis of 2000 Patients." Journal of Cardiothoracic Surgery. April 12, 2016. https://www.ncbi.nlm.nih.gov/pubmed/27068030

[19] Geka, Kyobu. "Effect of Autologous Platelet-Rich Plasma (PRP) in Cardiac Surgery." US National Library of Medicine National Institutes of Health. May 2001. https://www.ncbi.nlm.nih.gov/pubmed/11357304

Chapter 6

No Knee Joint Is an Island

Everything in your body is connected to everything else. We say that to our patients all the time—but what exactly do we mean? Perhaps the simplest explanation is that if I pinch your hand very hard, it will make tears come out of your eyes. You may think your hand and your eyes are not connected, but clearly, they are.

In the same way, treatments must consider the whole body. The physical-therapy recommendations for back injuries such as a herniated disc usually include a series of abdominal-muscle-strengthening exercises that, over time, will work to support the back.

The knee joint is just as complex as spinal joints. There are other elements that attach to and support it, including the anterior cruciate ligament, posterior cruciate ligament, and lateral and medial collateral ligaments. There's the quad muscle that attaches to the front of the knee joint, and the hamstring and calf muscles that are connected to the back. In short, a host of body parts come together to support the knee. To paraphrase John Donne's book about the human condition, no body part is an island.

In one way or another, everything (like everyone) depends on everything else. For that reason, when you want full func-tionality of a knee joint, it's important to consider that what's around it may need strengthening in order to support that joint. In rehabilitating the back, we don't just focus on the back. In rehabilitating the knee, we don't simply focus on the knee.

Rehabilitation is a significant component of recovery. We generally recommend it for patients in conjunction with one or more of the protocols, such as PRP and/or stem cell injections and Class 4 lasers, which will be featured in Chapter 7. It's vital to know which exercises and which gear are right for your particular injury and source of pain. Wise rehabilitation can mean the difference between a full recovery and something far less.

When there is evidence of a degenerative condition, misalignment and imbalance are often also involved. In such cases, we have to take care of not just the joint, but also the misalignment and imbalance. As we discussed in Chapter 1, knee decompression helps increase the crucial space inside the knee joint when it has diminished with age, often bringing along pain, immobility, and falls due to instability. What also happens is the unstable knees can buckle or misalign, putting abnormal pressure on the joint and facilitating the degenerative process.

Knee-decompression therapy uses motorized therapeutic equipment to gently open up the knee space and align the knee joint. As described in Chapter 1, the knee is filled with a lubricating, cushioning fluid (synovial fluid) that simply cannot circulate if there is no space for it to do so. Knee decompres-sion allows fluid to re-inhabit the knee as it did presurgery, pre-injury, or prior to other age-related issues. Even if you've been told you are "bone on bone," I encourage you to seek a second opinion from me. Often, I find that patients still have hope and we frequently help them avoid surgery using PRP therapy, stem cell injection, and knee-decompression therapy.

If the Brace Fits . . .

Because knee rehabilitation (techniques and machines) is not a one-size-fits-all proposition, it's important to consider the parameters of your specific injury or source of pain before embarking on a program. We offer a different type of reha-bilitation that is not the same as physical therapy.

We know that some of our patients travel great distances to get to our clinic for treatment, and extended rehab is not always possible. In those instances, following treatment, we might recommend braces—hinged, unhinged, or combination types—depending on the patients' needs (is the goal to walk around the block three times a week or play singles tennis every day?) and the extent of degeneration.

Another type of rehabilitation we endorse at our clinic is Rapid Release

Technology, or RRT. This therapy employs a device that delivers high-speed vibration (it feels like a massage) to break up scar tissue. If you have had an injury, you have scar tissue. Because scar tissue has no blood vessels and therefore receives no circulation, it can become brittle and constrictive, isolating nerves, limiting flexibility, reducing range of motion, and causing pain. RRT is used to break up scar tissue, which can help restore the knee.

Sometimes patients come to us proclaiming they've been on a knee-exercise regimen for a long time, possibly recommended by a personal trainer. While they may have gotten some relief, they say the pain returns when they stop exercising, or that it comes and goes. If random knee exercises were assigned to you—but not in conjunction with other protocols, such as the ones outlined in this book—they may be helping with the pain, but the relief is temporary and short lived. Probably, that pain is rooted in degenerative changes in the knee, which get worse every day. Routine exercises will not fix degeneration; they can only provide temporary relief. The problem must be confronted from all sides with a customized protocol to regenerate knee tissue. Without this type of therapy for the degenerative joint, the pain will often return.

Long after knee-replacement surgery, Brenda was still experiencing pain. She came to us to find out why.

"My knee still hurts," she said. She was surprised that her artificial knee *could* still hurt. She was deeply disappointed and had little hope that anything more could be done for her. Patients must understand that surgery doesn't come with a guaranteed result. If the surgery is not successful, the patient might even be left in worse condition than he or she was before the surgery.

When we asked Brenda precisely where it hurt, she pointed to muscles and ligaments around the knee. We explained to her that, while it might sound counterintuitive, even something as seemingly comprehensive as knee-replacement surgery might not fully resolve knee pain. A knee replacement must be balanced with muscle-strengthening work; we call this kind of rehabilitation "soft-tissue work." Soft tissue includes muscles, tendons, ligaments, and fascia, all of which need to be addressed for an optimal recovery.

In cases like Brenda's, we might also recommend PRP or stem cell injections to augment healing. With this kind of combined therapeutic effort, we can often greatly improve or eliminate knee pain. I used to turn away patients with artificial joints, believing nothing more could be done for them. But we have found that by treating the support structures around the knee joint, such as ligaments and muscles, we are able to help patients find tremendous improvement, even after knee replacement.

It's important to remember that our bodies comprise a lot of moving parts, and each part can be made up of yet more moving parts! Designing a custom, long-range plan that takes everything into account is the blueprint for success in relieving knee pain.

Chapter 7

How Class 4 Lasers Get Your Blood Flowing

As mentioned in previous chapters, we often recommend combined therapies for optimal results. These combina-tions may include stem cell injections, PRP injections, knee decompression, RRT, special supplements, and other forms of treatment we've explored. While each patient who comes to us in pain is thoroughly evaluated on an individual basis for knee, back, neck, or other joint issues, it's finding the right therapy "cocktail" that helps us achieve the best outcome for pain-free function and mobility.

Welcome to Class 4 laser therapy, a noninvasive, highly potent therapeutic tool to rapidly decrease the swelling and inflammation that are part of the pain cycle.

But first, here's a little bit about laser therapy in general.

In past years, the practice of laser therapy used what is called a "cold" laser. The cold laser—which is still used today in some practices—alleviated swelling and inflammation to a certain extent. In fact, I had good results using it on patients. But a cold laser is a low-level laser; some are barely more powerful than a bar-code scanner or laser pointer!

Class 4 lasers, sanctioned by the FDA in 2003, are much stronger and more advanced, and are considered today's standard of care. Class 4 lasers use penetrating heat to dilate blood vessels around an affected area to promote healing. The injured part of the body, to which the laser is applied, benefits from increased blood flow to the tissues. While scientists still don't agree about exactly how this works, lasers are thought to stimulate cells to produce more ATP, or cellular energy. The result is faster, improved healing time: Swelling and inflammation sometimes begin to subside within a matter of minutes.

I once had a patient who fell off a stool in a hospital and landed on his face while visiting a friend. Talk about iatrogenic (hospital-caused) injury! He came to me with neck pain and massive swelling and bruising on his face. I used Class 4 laser treatment, and we could see his swelling going down *as I was treating him!* Class 4 laser therapy can be a powerful treatment for both acute and chronic inflammation.

Unlike stem cell injections, which can travel to other parts of the body in need of healing, the Class 4 laser is designed to treat just one spot. This means we can do even more than aim it generally at a knee, elbow, or shoulder. It works with such precision that, if a patient tells us the *inside* of the knee hurts more—or the *back* of the knee, or the *left side* of the knee—we can apply the laser therapy directly to the area of pain. The intense heat the laser generates feels very good for chronic-knee-pain patients. It is one of the most popular therapy stations in our practice.

The Ideal Candidate

Unlike the other therapies we've addressed, which can be less effective for patients who are aged or have diseases like diabetes, Class 4 laser therapy succeeds with nearly every candidate who comes into our clinic and qualifies for it. If you have metal in your body—such as an artificial joint, plates and screws from a repaired fracture, or a pacemaker—laser therapy might not be appropriate, as the laser can cause the metal to overheat. In those circumstances, we would focus on the other available treatments.

Again, the best results are often achieved with a combina-tion of one, two, or more therapies. If you were to undergo Class 4 laser treatment for a knee injury, it might be combined with either stem cell or PRP therapy, or even both—along with four weeks of knee-decompression therapy.

The Class 4 laser is used widely in both the medical and veterinary professions and is a powerful tool in the healing process because it can alleviate swelling and inflammation, two big components of knee injuries. The Class 4 laser is so effec-tive that doctors who travel with Olympic athletes are known to take a laser device with them. Organizations including the World Health Organization, the American Physical Therapy Association, and the International Association for the Study of Pain have endorsed Class 4 laser therapy. But for us, the real proof is in the way our patients respond.

One of our patients, Jeff, was an active individual in his early seventies. He was the CEO of his own company and loved to play golf, which he found increasingly difficult to do because of a painful elbow. Jeff was a good candidate for stem cell therapy, so we introduced that course of treatment, gave it a chance to differentiate, and followed up with eight Class 4 laser treatments—lasting about ten minutes each— over four weeks. The stem cells need to be given a chance to work before being exposed to laser treatment, as there was a chance they could be destroyed by the concentration of heat. Upon completion of the two therapies, Jeff's elbow pain was completely gone and he looked forward to getting out on the links with friends as often as he wanted.

My personal experience with a Class 4 laser involved a bike accident that left me with full-blown, raging road rash on my arm (along with a dislocated shoulder). The skin destruction was the equivalent of a third-degree burn; layers of my skin were stripped off and the arm became infected. The pain was excruciating. While it may sound counterintuitive to introduce a Class 4 laser to a burn-type injury, my treatment helped me find total pain relief and rapid healing. My recovery would not have been the same without it.

Class 4 laser therapy is an important form of treatment in a comprehensive program for overcoming knee and other joint-related pain. Remember, not all laser treatments are the same. Many cold-laser therapies that are still offered by doctors are not powerful enough to deliver good results. Class 4 laser therapy can generate deep, penetrating heat to reduce inflammation, decrease pain, and restore function—at the speed of laser light!

Chapter 8

Should We Continue the Conversation? Questions to Ask Yourself

By now, you've read all the information we've presented about the surgery-free path to knee-pain relief. In considering a visit to our clinic, you may have asked yourself some impor-tant questions about your particular injury and pain—and you might be wondering if you are a candidate for Oklahoma Physical Medicine and the various drug-free solutions we offer.

Perhaps the number one question for you to consider, and for us to learn the answer to, is just how long you've been in pain. Has it been a few weeks? A few months? How about years—maybe to the point where you cannot remember what it was like *not* to be in pain?

While we always appreciate patients who come to us early—which can keep a small, more manageable problem from exploding into a huge one— many of our patients have indeed been living with pain and physical limitations for a long period of time. They've become habituated to it. You might say pain and the avoidance of more pain has become a way of life.

Maybe you're someone who cannot recall what it was like to go through your days and nights without pain. Perhaps you have adapted to chronic pain by giving up favorite things such as after-dinner walks, playing golf or tennis, or simple day-to-day activities such as playing with your grandchildren and even grocery shopping. Maybe your spouse has to drop you off right at the door of the grocery store because a walk through the parking lot, compounded by getting all the way through your shopping list, is just too much.

Possibly you've cut down on time with friends because of any physical activity involved. You and your spouse might be afraid to plan vacations because you're worried you won't be able to handle all that walking. Maybe you've moved your bedroom from upstairs to downstairs because you find it difficult to maneuver around your own home.

Ask yourself this: If you're already forfeiting these kinds of activities, how much more will you have to forgo in the future if you allow your condition to worsen rather than take steps to change it now?

During my nursing education, I worked at a skilled nursing facility. One of the residents to whom I was assigned was ninety-four years old. Each morning, because of her pain and resulting limitations, I had to help her out of bed and to the restroom, then wheel her to the dining room and put food in front of her. But it wasn't enough. I had to cut the food and feed her as well. It isn't hard to imagine that this woman had lived a full life at one point. But gradually, over the years, she'd lost function until she could not do simple things, like stand up, walk, and use the toilet. Most of us would love to live to be ninety-four—but is this the kind of life you look forward to as you age? Where do *you* see yourself in the next five years? Ten years? If you don't like what you see, you must do something about your pain now.

The next question you should ask yourself is, just how often does your pain occur? Do you get it once a month? Maybe a few times a month? Once a week? Chances are, if you're reading this book, your knee pain (or pain in another joint) occurs much more often than that, and again, it has impacted how you move through your life. We understand that chronic knee pain can affect those around you, too. What have your friends and family had to give up to accommodate your pain and immobility? Can you honestly say that you are the best wife, best husband, best parent, best caregiver to aging parents, or best friend you can be when you are in pain and suffering?

Probing more deeply into the problem—which helps us consider you a viable candidate for our practice—we also need to know what the pain feels like and what you are doing when it occurs. Is it there when you take a walk and more intense when you work out at the gym, for example? What happens when you get in or out of a car? Are you climbing the stairs when it starts, and do you postpone the climb until you've worked through the pain—if that's even possible? Because we take a team (doctors and clinicians) approach to healing, these answers and more help all of us determine if you are a good candidate for treatment, and, if so, what course of therapy will be the most beneficial.

The next question you may want to ask yourself is if you've been told you need surgery—and if you were told it's the only option. A point we have emphasized repeatedly is that surgery is—more often than not—*not* the only option. In fact, some patients come to us after surgery because they are still in pain. In most cases, they weren't told about all the alternatives.

We'd like to know if you've been on a medication prescribed for your condition for a month or more, and if you still feel the need for it. In Chapter 2, we pointed out that there are no "magic pills" to instantaneously stop pain and speed recovery from an injury, and that even the most seemingly benign over-the-counter medications can cause dangerous side effects. And let's face it, medication may work to mask pain for a while, but it never fixes the root cause of the problem.

Perhaps you've been told your age and the degeneration of your body is causing your knee pain—and if age is to blame, that "you simply have to live with it." But it doesn't have to be that way! Some of the therapies outlined in this book, including knee decompression—where we noninvasively open up knee space to allow lubricating synovial fluid to re-inhabit it—work extremely well to rejuvenate aging knees even in patients with advanced age.

It's true, we are living longer—much longer—and some experts say we are outliving our bodies, and wallets. But there is so much that can be done, years and years ahead of any final curtain, to bring back the pleasurable lifestyle and mobility you might have lost to pain.

A Step in Our Direction

We know that once you've made a decision that you may be a good candidate for our practice some degree of reluctance might still remain. What we offer is an alterna-tive to conventional thinking about drugs and surgery. You may achieve outstanding results with our therapies, but as human beings, we tend to gravitate toward the comfortable and familiar—things we already know. Effective or not, drugs and surgery are in our national lexicon, while stem cells, PRP therapy, knee decompression, and Class 4 lasers are not so much. Our goal is to change that. We also aim to change the kind of thinking people tend to fall back into, such as deciding to do nothing.

To that end, we sometimes ask people (especially men, as it is a prime topic) about their *cars*—that's right, their cars! Men tend to take better care of their cars than they do of themselves. As soon as a light illuminates on the dashboard, or you're driving and hear something that's not quite right, do you take the car to a mechanic? Chances are you do, because you know if you ignore the warning signs, the problem will only get worse. Then you might be faced with a bigger, more expensive issue—one that can become so bad that, over time, you may not be able to drive the car.

Our bodies work the same way. Pain is a warning light. If you avoid addressing injury and pain, you'll have the same results for your body as if you ignored a warning light on your car.

What about women? We mentioned earlier that women tend to be caregivers—putting everyone and everything ahead of their own well-being. Women take care of their husbands, their children, their parents, grandchildren, neighbors, and friends first. Is that you?

We talked about having a child who complains about ongoing pain. When that's the case, do you advise the child to continue to live with it because he or she has had it for a while, so it must be normal? Of course not! But when women's bodies are trying to tell them something, very often that message gets relegated to the back burner—maybe months and years behind everything else. But what happens when the pain gets to the point that it impedes doing what you do for everyone else, as it very well can?

Most patients suffer from degenerative conditions that get worse as they age. Your best chance of healing is right now—not tomorrow, not a month from now, and certainly not a year from now, as your body continues to degenerate. We strive to work with patients who are already experiencing advanced levels of pain and degeneration, but getting in early is always the best medicine.

Coming Aboard

When you contact us for an appointment, you might have some questions and concerns about what will take place. We try to make the process go as smoothly as possible. In order to do that, we will email you a welcome video with information about us and what you can expect. We'll also provide you with a *symptom survey,* a detailed questionnaire you'll fill out for our team of doctors and clinicians. This allows us to get a comprehensive look at what is going on to come up with an optimal treatment plan for you. It's good to fill out the survey and send it ahead of time, but you also can bring it with you to your appointment along with any imaging you may have for our staff to review. If you don't have imaging, we will use our digital x-ray and fluoroscopy equipment (Chapter 1) to obtain the most complete picture of your injury.

Most people are good historians when it comes to their pain. The combination of the symptom survey, imaging, and open communication between patient and doctor sets the stage for a great outcome.

What about Cost?

Insurance plans cover certain types of therapies, but most plans do not cover what we consider premium therapies. Though the use of stem cells and PRP in treatment modalities has been around now for decades—with proven, peer-reviewed results—these therapies do not fall within the list of treatments accepted by insurance companies. We have asked key representatives in the insurance industry why this is so, and the simple answer is that it has to do with lobbying and money. What we do enables patients to stop taking medication and to avoid surgery. This can make formidable pharmaceutical and health-care giants stand to lose money, and they are not going to take these changes sitting down.

Patients should expect to pay cash when they come to our clinic. We do offer different ways of financing treatment, including no-interest options and the possibility of in-office financing, which our staff is ready to discuss with you. We understand what you need and what you can afford are two different subjects. If a patient does not quality for one service, we have approximately thirty different treatment options that the patient may be able to afford. We want you to know we make every effort to make treatment attainable for everyone's budget.

It's time for you to take back the lifestyle you once had—the one you deserve!

Please contact us at 405-726-2727.

Are you ready to live pain-free? We're ready to help you get there!

www.ingramcontent.com/pod-product-compliance
Lightning Source LLC
Chambersburg PA
CBHW071444210326
41597CB00020B/3930